Dr. Royal Rife:

Healing Frequencies for Physical and Mental Balance

Table of contents

Dr. Royal Rife:...0

Table of contents.....................................1

Introduction 1

Chapter 1:...5

The Science of Sound...............................5

The Physics Behind Sound Waves.................5

How Sound Travels and Interacts with Matters
....8

Resonance and Its Effects on the Human Body
....11

Chapter 2:..13

The Body's Energy Systems 13

The Body's Energy Systems......................13

Health Beyond Matters 15

The Basics of Qi Energy 18

Impact of Energy Imbalance 20

Energy and Emotions..............................23

Chapter 3:..27

Ancient Traditions of Healing with Sound.......27

Ancient Uses of Sounds for Healing 27

Traditional Instruments and Practices 31

Cultural Variation 34

Qi, Sound, and Frequency 37

Chapter 4: 40

Modern Practices of Sound Healing 40

Rife Machines 41

Contemporary Sound Healing Techniques.....42

The Role of Music and Certain Frequencies ...45

PEMF Therapy Explained....................................48

Frequencies that Heal...54

At-Home PEMF Therapy 56

Qi Coils and Other Products 59

Chapter 5: The Future of Sound Healing........65

Potential Integration of Sound Healing into Maintaining Healthcare 66

Emerging Research 70

Chapter 6:...74

Practical Exercises...74

How to Implement PEMF Therapy at Home ...74

How to Apply Frequencies at Home 77

Implementing Healing Frequencies.................81

Meditation and Exercise....................................84

Conclusion 90

Imprint...93

Introduction

Did you know that cat's purrs are more than just a sign of content? Cats purr at a certain frequency (25-150 Hertz). Coincidentally, this is also the frequency range that promotes the healing of broken bones, joint and tendon repair, and wound healing. With this scientifically proven fact right in front of us, how come there are so limited studies on this subject?

The power of sound and vibrations has long been recognized and utilized in ancient cultures for healing and rejuvenation. From the rhythmic beats of drums to the enchanting melodies of flutes, ancient civilizations around the world understood the profound impact that sound could have on the human body, mind, and spirit.

The connection between sound and the human body is profound and multifaceted. Sound, as a form of energy, has the ability to influence and interact with various physiological and psychological processes within the human body.

At a fundamental level, sound is perceived by the ears through a complex mechanism involving the outer, middle, and inner ear. Sound waves travel through the air or other mediums, causing vibrations in the ear canal. These vibrations are then transmitted to the eardrum and subsequently to the tiny hair cells in the cochlea, which convert them into electrical signals that are sent to the brain for interpretation.

Beyond the auditory system, sound can have a broader impact on the body. It is worth noting that the human body itself is composed of vibrating matter. Every organ, tissue, and cell in the body has its own unique frequency or resonance. When exposed to external sound vibrations, these internal structures can be influenced and respond accordingly.

Studies have shown that certain frequencies and vibrations can have a direct impact on the body's systems. For instance, lower frequencies, such as those found in deep bass tones, have been found to stimulate the production of endorphins, which are natural pain-relieving and mood-enhancing substances. On the other hand, higher frequencies, like the delicate sounds of harps or flutes, can induce a state of relaxation and calmness, reducing stress and anxiety.

The connection between sound and the body is not limited to the auditory experience alone. Vibrations can be felt and experienced throughout the body. This is exemplified in practices like sound massage or sound therapy, where instruments like singing bowls, tuning forks, or gongs are placed directly on or near the body. The vibrations produced by these instruments are believed to resonate with the body's tissues and energy centers, promoting relaxation, releasing tension, and restoring balance.

Moreover, the emotional and psychological impact of sound on the human body should not be underestimated. Music, for example, has the ability to evoke powerful emotions, elicit memories, and affect mood. Certain sounds or melodies can uplift the spirit, inspire motivation, or provide solace during challenging times. The connection between sound and emotions is deeply intertwined, and the power of sound to influence our emotional well-being is a subject of ongoing exploration and research.

The human body is intricate and far-reaching. From the physiological processes involved in hearing to the broader impact on biological rhythms, emotions, and overall well-being, sound has a profound influence on various aspects of our being. The exploration of sound as a therapeutic tool and the recognition of its potential to promote healing, relaxation, and rejuvenation continues to expand our understanding of this remarkable connection between sound and the human body.

Here, we will explore how ancient civilizations discovered and implemented these sounds and frequencies, how such traditional practices are modernized, and, most importantly, how you can implement these practices and reap their many benefits.

Chapter 1:
The Science of Sound

Let us start from the beginning. We can hear the world around us, but not many people actually know how sounds work, much less so about how they affect our bodies. We will talk about that here.

The Physics Behind Sound Waves

Sound is a mechanical wave, meaning it requires a medium, such as air, water, or solids, to traverse through. It consists of differences in pressure and displacement that travel through the medium in the form of longitudinal waves. Simply put, sound waves travel similarly to water waves.

Sound waves are characterized by several key properties. The frequency of a sound wave is the number of vibrations or cycles it achieves in a second. It is measured in Hz or Hertz.

Frequency determines the pitch of a sound, with higher frequencies associated with higher-pitched sounds and lower frequencies associated with lower-pitched sounds. For example, the sound of a high-pitched whistle has a higher frequency than the sound of a low-pitched drum.

Another important property is amplitude, which is how far the particles in the medium are displaced from their original position which results from the passing of sound waves.

Amplitude, another important property, refers to the maximum displacement of particles in the medium from their original position as the sound wave passes through. Amplitude determines the loudness or intensity of a sound, with greater amplitude corresponding to a louder sound and smaller amplitude corresponding to a softer sound.

The relationship between frequency and wavelength is crucial in understanding sound waves. Wavelength is the distance between two repeated patterns in a single phase. Simply put, imagine the top of two mountains of exactly the same shape. The distance between the top of those two mountains is the wavelength. The wavelength is inversely proportional to the frequency, meaning that as the frequency increases, the wavelength decreases, and vice versa.

Sound waves can also undergo reflection, refraction, diffraction, and interference. Reflection occurs when sound waves bounce off a surface, like an echo bouncing off a wall. Refraction refers to the bending of sound waves as they pass through different mediums with varying densities, causing changes in their direction. Diffraction refers to the bending and spreading out of sound waves around obstacles or through openings. Interference occurs when two or more sound waves overlap, resulting in either constructive interference (amplification) or destructive interference (cancellation) depending on the relative phase of the waves.

How Sound Travels and Interacts with Matters

Sound travels through matter as a result of the interaction between sound waves and the particles or molecules present in the medium. The transmission of sound involves a series of intricate processes that depend on the characteristics of the medium itself.

When a sound is produced, it generates vibrations or disturbances in the air, water, or solid material around it. These vibrations create a pressure wave that compresses and rarefies the particles or molecules of the medium.

When a sound wave passes through the air, it causes the air particles to oscillate back and forth, transferring energy from one particle to the next. The particles themselves do not move along with the sound wave; instead, they vibrate around their equilibrium positions. This is why sound waves in gases are referred to as longitudinal waves.

In liquids, such as water, sound waves also propagate as longitudinal waves, but with a higher density of particles compared to gases.

As sound travels through water, it causes the water molecules to oscillate, transmitting the sound energy from molecule to molecule. The denser arrangement of particles in liquids allows sound waves to travel at a faster speed compared to gases.

In solids, sound waves can travel as both longitudinal and transverse waves. In longitudinal waves, similar to gases and liquids, particles vibrate parallel to the direction of wave propagation. In transverse waves, particles oscillate perpendicular to the direction of wave propagation. This dual nature of sound waves in solids is due to the interconnected lattice structure of solid materials. The particles in a solid are closely packed and firmly connected, allowing sound waves to propagate efficiently through the solid medium.

The speed at which sound travels through a medium depends on various factors, including the density and elasticity of the material. Generally, sound travels faster in denser and more elastic materials. For example, sound travels faster through solids than through liquids, and faster through liquids than through gases. This is because the particles in denser materials are closer together, facilitating faster energy transfer.

When sound waves encounter different materials or encounter changes in the characteristics of the medium, they can undergo various interactions. Reflection occurs when sound waves bounce off a surface, such as an echo bouncing off a wall. Refraction happens when sound waves change direction as they pass from one medium to another with different densities. Diffraction occurs when sound waves bend or spread out as they encounter obstacles or pass through openings. Absorption takes place when sound waves transfer their energy to the particles of the medium, resulting in a decrease in the sound's intensity.

Resonance and Its Effects on the Human Body

Resonance is a phenomenon that occurs when an object or a system is exposed to an external force or stimulus at its natural frequency, causing it to vibrate with increased amplitude. In the context of the human body, resonance can have various effects and implications.

The human body consists of numerous structures, tissues, and organs, each with its own unique natural frequencies of vibration. These frequencies are determined by factors such as size, shape, and elasticity of the body parts. When exposed to external vibrations or sound waves that match or closely align with these natural frequencies, resonance can occur.

One example of resonance in the body is the vibration of vocal cords during speech or singing. When air passes through the vocal cords, they vibrate at their natural frequency, producing sound waves that can be heard as speech or singing. The resonance of the vocal cords amplifies and enhances the sound produced, allowing us to communicate effectively.

Resonance can also be observed in the interaction between sound waves and various organs or body cavities. For instance, the resonance of sound in the chest cavity can enhance the sound produced by the lungs and heart, contributing to the richness and quality of certain sounds during auscultation or medical examinations.

Furthermore, resonance has been explored in the field of sound therapy and healing modalities. Instruments like singing bowls, gongs, and tuning forks are used to produce specific frequencies and vibrations that resonate with different parts of the body. The theory behind these practices suggests that the vibrations created by these instruments can resonate with and influence the body's tissues, cells, and energy centers, promoting relaxation, balance, and overall well-being.

Resonance is a complex phenomenon, and its effects on the body depend on various factors, including the intensity, duration, and frequency of the stimulus, as well as the individual's physiological characteristics and sensitivity. Further research is still needed to

fully understand and harness the potential
benefits of resonance in therapeutic
applications.

Chapter 2:

The Body's Energy Systems

In the last chapter, we talked about how exactly sound affects our bodies. In this chapter, we will go further beyond – more than what big pharma wants you to know. The lessons you take from this chapter stems from studies done by ancient civilizations (more on that in the next chapter), and understanding them is key to understanding how your body truly works.

The Body's Energy Systems

The human body is not only composed of physical matter but also intricately connected to subtle energy systems. These energy systems, found in various cultures and healing traditions worldwide, provide a framework for understanding the subtle aspects of our being and their influence on our overall well-being.

Two prominent examples of these energy systems are chakras and meridians.

Chakras, originating from ancient Indian spiritual traditions and now widely recognized in various spiritual and healing practices, are centers of energy located along the central channel of the body. There are 7 main chakras, each connected to a certain physical, emotional, and spiritual part of our being.

These energy centers are believed to influence our vitality, emotions, thought patterns, and spiritual development. The chakras are often depicted as spinning wheels or lotus flowers, representing the flow and balance of energy within them.

Meridians, on the other hand, are energy pathways recognized in traditional Chinese medicine. They form an intricate network that connects different parts of the body, organs, and acupoints. It is believed that Qi, the vital energy, flows through these meridians, supporting the functioning of the organs and maintaining overall health. Acupuncture and acupressure are techniques used to influence the flow of Qi within the meridians, aiming to restore balance and promote well-being.

These subtle energy systems provide a holistic understanding of the interconnectedness between our physical, emotional, mental, and spiritual aspects. They offer a perspective that goes beyond the purely physical and acknowledges the presence of subtle energies and their influence on our well-being. By working with these energy systems, it is believed that we can enhance our vitality, release blockages, and promote a sense of balance and harmony within ourselves.

Health Beyond Matters

Chakras and meridians, as subtle energy systems within the human body, are believed to play significant roles in supporting overall health and well-being. While their existence and mechanisms may be challenging to measure and quantify in scientific terms, many individuals and practitioners have reported experiencing positive effects when working with these energy systems. Here are some ways in which chakras and meridians are thought to contribute to health and well-being:

- Balancing and harmonizing energy: Chakras and meridians are considered to be responsible for the flow of energy throughout the body. When these energy systems are in a state of balance and harmony, it is believed to support optimal physical, emotional, and mental functioning. By working with techniques such as meditation, breathwork, yoga, or energy healing practices, individuals may seek to clear blockages and restore the smooth and balanced flow of energy within these systems.

- Enhancing vitality and energy levels: It is believed that the balanced flow of energy through the chakras and meridians contributes to increased vitality and overall energy levels. When energy flows freely, it can support the body's natural healing processes, boost the immune system, and promote a sense of vitality and aliveness.

- Supporting emotional well-being: Different chakras are associated with specific emotions and psychological states. For example, the heart chakra is often linked to love, compassion, and emotional balance, while the solar plexus chakra is associated with personal power and self-esteem. By working with these energy centers, individuals may aim to cultivate emotional awareness, release emotional blockages, and promote emotional well-being.

- Facilitating spiritual growth and awareness: Chakras, in particular, are closely connected to spiritual development and consciousness. For instance, the third eye and crown chakras are associated with intuition, spiritual connection, and a heightened state of consciousness. Practices like meditation, visualization, and energy healing can be used to activate and align these chakras, supporting spiritual growth and deepening one's sense of connection to the divine or higher self.
- Regulating and balancing the body's systems: Meridians, as recognized in traditional Chinese medicine, are closely linked to the body's organs and their functions. The flow of Qi through the meridians is believed to influence the functioning of the organs and promote overall health. By stimulating specific acupoints along the meridians, for example, through acupuncture or

acupressure, it is thought that balance can be restored, promoting the body's natural healing mechanisms and supporting various physiological processes.

These energy systems are not isolated from other aspects of health and well-being. They are interconnected with physical, emotional, and mental factors, and should be considered as part of a holistic approach to well-being.

While the scientific understanding of these energy systems is still evolving, many individuals find value in exploring and working with chakras and meridians as complementary practices to support their overall health, self-awareness, and personal growth.

The Basics of Qi Energy

Qi, also spelled as "Chi" or "Ki," is a fundamental concept in traditional Chinese culture and philosophy. It is often translated as "vital energy" or "life force." Qi is believed to be a pervasive and dynamic energy that flows through all living beings and the natural world, connecting everything in the universe.

In traditional Chinese medicine, Qi is considered an essential element for maintaining health and well-being. It is believed that when Qi is balanced and flowing harmoniously, the body is in a state of good health, both physically and mentally. On the other hand, disruptions or imbalances in Qi can lead to illness and disharmony.

The concept of Qi is often described using metaphorical terms, such as the flow of a river or the movement of air. It is said to circulate through channels or pathways in the body called meridians. These meridians form a network that connects the organs, tissues and vital energy centers known as acupoints. By stimulating specific acupoints, it is believed that the flow of Qi can be influenced and restored to achieve balance and health.

Qi is understood to have different qualities or aspects, which include Yin and Yang. Yin represents the more passive, feminine, and nourishing aspects, while Yang represents the active, masculine, and transformative aspects. It is believed that maintaining a harmonious balance between Yin and Yang within the body is vital for overall well-being.

While the concept of Qi is deeply rooted in traditional Chinese culture and philosophy, it can be challenging to describe or quantify using scientific terms. It does not have a direct equivalent in Western scientific understanding. However, some aspects of Qi can be related to physiological processes such as the circulation of blood, the movement of nerve impulses, and the exchange of energy within cells.

In recent years, there has been growing interest in exploring the concept of Qi from a scientific perspective. Researchers have studied various phenomena related to Qi, such as bioelectric fields, electromagnetic energy, and the effects of mind-body practices like Qigong and Tai Chi on health and well-being. While scientific investigations are ongoing, the understanding of Qi in the context of traditional Chinese medicine remains rooted in ancient philosophy and holistic perspectives.

Impact of Energy Imbalance

Imbalances in the energy systems, such as chakras and meridians, are believed to have a significant impact on both physical and mental health. According to various traditional healing systems and holistic approaches, these imbalances can manifest in different ways and contribute to a range of health issues. Here are some ways in which imbalances in the energy systems may affect physical and mental well-being:

1. Physical Health:

   - Disrupted organ function: In traditional Chinese medicine, meridians are closely linked to specific organs. Imbalances or blockages in the meridians may disrupt the flow of energy to the corresponding organs, potentially affecting their function and leading to physical symptoms or diseases.

   - Weakened immune system: Imbalances in the energy systems can impact the body's overall vitality and immune response. When the energy flow is hindered or deficient, the body's ability to fight off infections, heal injuries, and maintain optimal health may be compromised.

- Physical pain and discomfort: Imbalances in the energy systems can contribute to physical pain or discomfort. For example, blockages in certain meridians or imbalances in specific chakras may be associated with localized pain or sensations in corresponding areas of the body.

2. Mental and Emotional Well-being:

- Emotional disturbances: Each chakra is associated with specific emotions and psychological states. Imbalances in the chakras can lead to emotional disturbances such as anxiety, depression, anger, or a lack of emotional balance and stability.

- Mental fog or confusion: When the energy flow is disrupted or stagnant, it may impact mental clarity and cognitive function. This can manifest as mental fog, difficulty concentrating, or a sense of confusion.

- Imbalanced moods and behavior: Imbalances in the energy systems can contribute to mood swings, irritability, or behavioral patterns that are out of alignment with one's usual state of being.

It's important to note that imbalances in the energy systems are often considered within a holistic context, taking into account physical, emotional, and mental aspects as interconnected. The impact of imbalances can vary among individuals, and specific symptoms or experiences may differ. Additionally, it is crucial to consider other factors such as lifestyle, environment, and underlying health conditions when addressing imbalances and seeking to restore harmony to the energy systems.

Various practices, such as energy healing modalities, acupuncture, yoga, meditation, and breathwork, aim to rebalance the energy systems and address imbalances. By restoring the flow of energy and promoting harmony within the energy systems, it is believed that physical and mental well-being can be improved, and the body's natural healing processes can be supported.

While the understanding and interpretation of these energy systems are rooted in traditional philosophies and holistic approaches, it's important to approach them with an open mind and consider them complementary to conventional medical care. Seeking guidance from qualified practitioners can provide valuable insights and support in addressing imbalances and promoting overall health and well-being.

Energy and Emotions

The connection between energy and emotions is a fascinating aspect of human experience. While emotions are often understood as subjective feelings and experiences, they also have an energetic component that can be perceived and influenced.

1. Energetic Nature of Emotions: Emotions are not solely confined to the realm of thoughts and feelings. They also generate an energetic charge within the

body. This energetic aspect can be experienced as sensations, vibrations, or shifts in the body's energy field. Different emotions are associated with varying energetic qualities. For instance, joy and love are often described as uplifting and expansive, while anger and fear may feel contracting or constricting.

2. Energy Flow and Emotions: Emotions are closely tied to the flow of energy within the body. When emotions arise, they can affect the movement and distribution of energy. For example, a surge of excitement might result in increased energy and heightened sensations, while sadness or grief may be accompanied by a sense of heaviness or low energy. Conversely, the flow of energy can also influence emotions. Practices such as deep breathing, movement, or energy healing techniques aim to regulate and balance the energy flow, which can have a positive impact on emotional well-being.

3. Emotional Imprints: Emotions can leave imprints in the body's energy field. Intense or prolonged emotional experiences, particularly those

associated with trauma or stress, can create energetic patterns or blockages. These imprints can linger in the body and contribute to the development of emotional patterns, behavioral tendencies, and even physical symptoms. By working with energy healing or therapeutic modalities, it is believed that these imprints can be released or harmonized, supporting emotional healing and well-being.

4. Energy Awareness and Emotional Regulation: Developing an awareness of one's energy can enhance emotional regulation and self-awareness. By tuning into the energetic aspect of emotions, individuals can gain insights into the subtle shifts and patterns within their emotional landscape. This awareness allows for greater recognition, acceptance, and understanding of emotions, promoting emotional intelligence and the ability to respond skillfully to different emotional states.

5. Influence of External Energy: The energetic qualities of emotions are not limited to an individual's internal experience. Emotions can also influence

and interact with the energy of others and the environment. Have you ever noticed how a tense or joyful atmosphere can impact your own emotional state? This interplay between individual and collective energy is significant and highlights the importance of creating supportive and nurturing environments for emotional well-being.

While the connection between energy and emotions is recognized in various healing traditions, it is essential to approach it with an open and integrative mindset. Western scientific frameworks may not fully explain the energetic aspects of emotions, but the lived experiences of individuals and the benefits reported from practices like energy healing, meditation, or breathwork highlight the potential of working with energy to positively impact emotional well-being.

Chapter 3:

Ancient Traditions of Healing with Sound

In many indigenous cultures, sound, and vibrations were believed to be interconnected with the natural world and the divine. They recognized that everything in the universe, including human beings, is composed of energy and vibrates at specific frequencies. By harnessing specific sounds and vibrations, they sought to restore balance and harmony within the individual and the surrounding environment. This chapter is a history lesson about how humanity has come to understand the healing powers of sound.

Ancient Uses of Sounds for Healing

Ancient civilizations recognized the profound power of sound for healing and incorporated it into their practices and rituals. Across various cultures and time periods, sound was believed to possess transformative qualities and the ability to restore balance and harmony within the body, mind, and spirit. Here are some examples of how ancient civilizations used sound for healing:

- Ancient Egypt: The ancient Egyptians used sound in their healing temples known as "Sleep Temples." These temples were dedicated to the god Imhotep, who was considered the god of healing. Healing rituals involved chanting, music, and the recitation of specific incantations or spells. The Egyptians believed that the vibrations created by sound had the power to align the individual with the divine and facilitate healing.
- Ancient Greece: In ancient Greece, music and sound were integral to the healing practices of renowned figures such as Pythagoras and Hippocrates. Pythagoras believed that music could harmonize the body and soul, and he developed the concept of the "Music of the Spheres," which stated that the celestial bodies emitted musical tones that influenced human well-being. Hippocrates, often referred to as the father of medicine,

used music as part of his therapeutic approach to balance the body's humor and promote healing.

- Ancient India: The ancient Indian civilization had a deep understanding of the power of sound and vibration. The practice of Nada Yoga, or the yoga of sound, was developed to harness the transformative qualities of sound for healing and spiritual growth. Mantras, sacred chants, and the recitation of specific Sanskrit syllables were employed to activate specific energy centers, promote balance, and purify the mind. The use of specific musical scales, known as "ragas," was also believed to have a therapeutic effect on different aspects of the body and mind.

- Ancient China: Traditional Chinese medicine incorporated sound healing as part of its holistic approach. The Chinese recognized the vital connection between sound, emotions, and organs in the body. They developed the Five Element Theory, which correlated specific sounds and musical tones with various organs and emotions. Sound healing practices, such as using specific instruments like the guqin or qigong exercises involving vocalization, were employed to restore harmony and balance within the body.

- Indigenous Cultures: Many indigenous cultures around the world have long-standing traditions of using sound for healing. Shamanic practices often involve the use of drums, rattles, singing, and chanting to induce altered states of consciousness and facilitate healing. These practices were believed to create a bridge between the human and spirit realms, allowing for energetic and spiritual healing.
- Native American cultures: also recognized the power of sound for healing and rejuvenation. Shamans and medicine people would utilize drums, rattles, and sacred chants in their ceremonies and rituals. These sounds were believed to invoke the spirits and establish a connection with the divine, facilitating healing at both the individual and community levels. The rhythmic beats of the drums, in particular, were thought to induce trance-like states, allowing individuals to access deeper levels of consciousness and tap into their innate healing abilities.

These examples highlight the reverence and understanding that ancient civilizations had for the power of sound in healing. Sound was seen as a sacred and integral part of their healing practices, aimed at restoring balance and promoting well-being on multiple levels. While the specific techniques and rituals varied across cultures, the underlying belief in the transformative and harmonizing qualities of sound remained consistent.

Today, we can draw inspiration from these ancient practices and integrate them into modern sound healing modalities. As we explore and embrace the ancient wisdom of sound, we have the opportunity to reconnect with this powerful healing tool and incorporate it into our own journeys of physical, emotional, and spiritual well-being.

Traditional Instruments and Practices

Traditional instruments and practices have been used across cultures for centuries as powerful tools for healing, meditation, and spiritual connection. These ancient traditions have withstood the test of time and continue to be valued and practiced in various forms around the world. Let's explore some of these traditional instruments and practices:

- Singing Bowls: Singing bowls originated in the Himalayan region, particularly in Tibet, Nepal, and Bhutan. These bowls are made of metal, typically a combination of copper and other metals. When the rim of the bowl is rubbed with a mallet, it produces a resonant and soothing sound. Singing bowls are often used in meditation and sound healing practices to induce relaxation, balance energy, and create a harmonious atmosphere.
- Chanting: Chanting is a practice of repetitive vocalization of sacred sounds, words, or phrases. It is found in various religious and spiritual traditions, such as Gregorian chants in Christianity, Vedic chants in Hinduism, or Buddhist chants like "Om Mani Padme Hum." Chanting serves to focus the mind, evoke a meditative state, and connect with the divine. The rhythmic vibrations of chanting can have a calming and centering effect on the practitioner.

- Drumming: Drumming is a universal practice found in cultures worldwide. The rhythmic beats and vibrations of drums have a profound impact on the mind, body, and spirit. Drumming has been used for ceremonial purposes, healing rituals, and community gatherings. The steady rhythm of the drum can induce trance-like states, facilitate emotional release, and promote a sense of unity and connectedness.
- Didgeridoo: The didgeridoo is a traditional wind instrument originating from Indigenous Australian cultures. Made from a hollowed-out tree trunk, the didgeridoo produces a distinctively deep and resonant sound. Playing the didgeridoo involves a continuous circular breathing technique, which has been shown to have therapeutic benefits for respiratory health and relaxation. The low-frequency vibrations of the didgeridoo can create a calming and grounding effect.
- Gongs: Gongs are large, metallic percussion instruments with a rich and complex sounds. They have been used in East Asian cultures, particularly in

China and Indonesia, for spiritual and healing purposes. The deep and resonant tones of gongs are believed to clear energy blockages, stimulate circulation, and induce deep relaxation. Gong baths, where multiple gongs are played simultaneously, have gained popularity as immersive sound healing experiences.

- Flutes: Various types of flutes are found in indigenous cultures across the globe. The Native American flute, for example, is known for its melodic and soulful sound. Playing the flute can have a soothing and meditative effect, promoting relaxation and introspection. The breath required to play the flute connects the player with their inner rhythm and can facilitate a sense of calm and presence.

These traditional instruments and practices offer unique sonic qualities and vibrational frequencies that resonate with the human body and spirit. They provide avenues for self-expression, introspection, and healing. Whether through the enchanting sound of a singing bowl, the rhythmic beat of a drum, or the melodic chant of sacred words, these traditional instruments and practices invite us to connect with our inner selves, commune with the divine, and tap into the healing potential of sound.

Incorporating these traditional instruments and practices into our lives can enhance our well-being, promote relaxation, and foster a deeper connection to ourselves and the world around us. Their enduring presence reminds us of the timeless wisdom and transformative power of sound in our journey toward balance, harmony, and spiritual growth.

Cultural Variation

Cultural variations in sound healing practices reflect the diverse beliefs, traditions, and approaches to well-being found around the world. These practices highlight the unique ways in which different cultures harness the power of sound for healing, spiritual connection, and personal transformation. Let's explore some cultural variations in sound healing practices:

- Indian Classical Music: In India, the ancient practice of Nada Yoga, the yoga of sound, has been used for centuries to achieve spiritual and physical well-being. Indian classical music, with its intricate melodies and rhythms, is believed to have a profound impact on the mind, body, and emotions. Ragas, specific musical scales associated with different times of the day or emotional states, are used to evoke specific moods and stimulate energy centers in the body.

- Japanese Shakuhachi Meditation: The shakuhachi is a traditional bamboo flute used in Zen Buddhist meditation in Japan. Playing the shakuhachi involves long, meditative breaths and intentional blowing techniques. The haunting and ethereal sounds of the shakuhachi are used to induce a state of deep relaxation, mindfulness, and contemplation.

- Aboriginal Dreamtime Healing: Indigenous Australian cultures have a deep connection to the land and use sound in their healing practices. The didgeridoo, a traditional wind instrument, is played as part of Dreamtime healing rituals. The vibrations and rhythmic patterns of the didgeridoo are believed to connect individuals with the spirit world, clear energy blockages, and restore harmony and balance.

- Peruvian Icaros: In the shamanic traditions of the Peruvian Amazon, healing songs called Icaros are used during Ayahuasca ceremonies. These melodic chants are believed to invoke spiritual entities and create a sacred space for healing and transformation. The Icaros guide participants through their inner journey, helping them navigate emotions, release energetic blockages, and reconnect with their true selves.
- African Drumming and Dance: Across the African continent, drumming and dance are integral to spiritual ceremonies, community gatherings, and healing rituals. The pulsating rhythms of the drums synchronize the heartbeat and create a collective energy that promotes a sense of unity, celebration, and spiritual connection. African drumming and dance allow individuals to release emotions, enter trance-like

states, and connect with ancestral spirits.

- Tibetan Buddhist Chanting: Tibetan Buddhism incorporates a rich tradition of chanting, often accompanied by various instruments like bells, cymbals, and horns. Mantras, such as the famous "Om Mani Padme Hum," are repeated to invoke compassion and wisdom. The vibrations created by the chanting are believed to purify the mind, balance energies, and cultivate a state of inner peace.

These examples represent just a fraction of the cultural variations in sound healing practices around the world. Each culture brings its unique perspectives, instruments, rituals, and beliefs about the healing power of sound. These practices demonstrate the deep connection between sound, spirituality, and well-being within different cultural contexts.

Exploring and honoring cultural variations in sound healing practices can broaden our understanding of the transformative potential of sound and deepen our appreciation for the diverse ways in which sound is used to promote healing and spiritual growth. It reminds us of the richness and wisdom that different cultures offer and encourages us to embrace and learn from these traditions to enhance our own well-being and foster cross-cultural appreciation.

Qi, Sound, and Frequency

In the context of traditional Chinese medicine and philosophy, there is a connection between Qi and sound and frequency. Sound and frequency are considered to be manifestations of Qi and are believed to have an impact on the flow and balance of Qi within the body.

In traditional Chinese medicine, different sounds are associated with specific organs and their corresponding meridians. It is believed that vocalizing certain sounds or tones can stimulate and harmonize the flow of Qi in those organs and meridians. These practices are often incorporated into therapeutic techniques like Qigong and sound healing.

Additionally, sound and vibration are seen as powerful tools for influencing Qi and promoting well-being. The use of specific frequencies, such as those produced by musical instruments, singing bowls, or tuning forks, is believed to have a resonating effect on the body's Qi and energy centers. The vibrations produced by these sounds are thought to help balance and restore the flow of Qi, supporting health and healing processes.

Furthermore, the practice of mindful listening and awareness of sound can be used to cultivate Qi. By focusing on and appreciating the subtle vibrations and frequencies in our environment, it is believed that we can enhance our connection to universal energy and promote a sense of harmony within ourselves.

Chapter 4:

Modern Practices of Sound Healing

In recent years, there has been a notable resurgence of interest in healing frequencies and their potential therapeutic benefits. As people search for alternative and holistic approaches to health and well-being, the power of sound and vibrations has once again captured the attention of individuals and practitioners alike.

Advancements in technology have also contributed to the resurgence of interest in healing frequencies. With the widespread availability of smartphones, tablets, and other portable devices, accessing and experiencing sound therapy has become more accessible than ever. Mobile applications and online platforms offer a wide range of sound therapy options, including guided meditations, binaural beats, and solfeggio frequency playlists, enabling individuals to incorporate these healing frequencies into their daily routines and self-care practices.

In this chapter, we will explore the many ways that sound healing is implemented in modern times.

Rife Machines

Rife machines, also known as Rife frequency generators or Rife devices, are electronic devices that were originally developed in the 1930s by Royal Raymond Rife, a prominent American inventor, and researcher. Rife machines were designed with the aim of using specific frequencies to treat various diseases and health conditions.

Royal Rife believed that every disease has a specific frequency at which it vibrates, and by exposing the body to that particular frequency, the disease-causing organisms or cells could be destroyed or neutralized. He conducted extensive research and claimed to have discovered specific frequencies that could target and eliminate various pathogens, including bacteria, viruses, and even cancer cells.

The Rife machine operates by generating electromagnetic frequencies that are then delivered to the body through electrodes or other means of transmission. It is based on the principle of resonance, where the targeted cells or organisms absorb the energy of a specific frequency, leading to their destruction. Rife believed that this approach could provide a non-invasive and potentially effective method for treating a wide range of ailments.

Over the years, Rife machines have undergone various modifications and improvements. Today, there are numerous models available in the market, ranging from basic frequency generators to more sophisticated devices with additional features. Some modern Rife machines may include other therapeutic modalities, such as pulsed electromagnetic field (PEMF) therapy or light therapy, to enhance their effectiveness.

Proponents of Rife machines claim that they can be used to address various health conditions, including infections, Lyme disease, arthritis, chronic pain, and even certain types of cancer.

Contemporary Sound Healing Techniques

Contemporary sound healing techniques, such as binaural beats, isochronic tones, and Solfeggio frequencies, have gained popularity for their potential to promote relaxation, enhance mental focus, and support overall well-being. These techniques harness the power of specific sound frequencies to create desired effects in the brain and body. Let's take a look at each one of them:

1. Binaural Beats: Binaural beats involve playing two slightly different frequencies simultaneously, one in each ear, to create a perceived third frequency. This phenomenon occurs in the brain and is believed to influence brainwave activity. For example, when a frequency of 200 Hz is played in one ear and 210 Hz in the other, the brain perceives a binaural beat of 10 Hz, which corresponds to the alpha brainwave state associated with relaxation and creativity. Binaural beats are often used to induce specific mental states, such as relaxation, focus, meditation, or sleep.

2. Isochronic Tones: Similar to binaural beats, isochronic tones utilize rhythmic pulses of sound at specific frequencies. Unlike binaural beats, isochronic tones do not require headphones and can be heard through speakers. The distinct pulses of sound are thought to entrain the brainwaves to the desired frequency, promoting mental and emotional states. Isochronic tones are known for their effectiveness in supporting relaxation, concentration, stress reduction, and sleep enhancement.

3. Solfeggio Frequencies: The Solfeggio frequencies are a set of ancient musical frequencies that date back to the medieval period. They are believed to have specific healing properties and were used in sacred chants and hymns. The Solfeggio scale has six very specific frequencies of 396 Hz, 417 Hz, 528 Hz, 639 Hz, 741 Hz, and 852 Hz. Each frequency is associated with different intentions, such as releasing fear and guilt, facilitating change, promoting love and compassion, enhancing communication, awakening intuition,

and promoting spiritual enlightenment. Solfeggio frequencies are often used in sound healing practices, meditation, and personal development.

Contemporary sound healing techniques like binaural beats, isochronic tones, and Solfeggio frequencies can be experienced through various mediums, including recorded audio tracks, specialized apps, or sound healing sessions. They are often used in combination with other sound healing modalities, such as guided meditations, sound baths, or energy healing practices, to enhance their effects and create a more immersive healing experience.

These sound healing techniques offer individuals an accessible and versatile approach to enhance relaxation, focus, and well-being. Integrating these techniques into a self-care routine or seeking guidance from qualified practitioners can provide opportunities for personal exploration and self-discovery on the journey of healing and personal growth.

The Role of Music and Certain Frequencies

Music and specific frequencies play a significant role in promoting physical and mental balance. Sound and music have a profound effect on our physiology and psychology, and they can be used intentionally to support our well-being. Here are some ways in which music and specific frequencies contribute to promoting balance:

- Relaxation and Stress Reduction: Music has the power to evoke emotions and induce a relaxation response in the body. Slow-tempo music with gentle melodies and harmonies can activate the parasympathetic nervous system, reducing stress hormones and promoting a state of relaxation. Soft, soothing sounds can help slow down heart rate, lower blood pressure, and release muscle tension, facilitating a sense of calm and tranquility.
- Mood Enhancement and Emotional Well-being: Different types of music can elicit various emotional responses. Upbeat, joyful music can boost mood

and increase feelings of happiness and positivity. Slow, melodic music can evoke introspection and a sense of peacefulness. By listening to music that resonates with our emotions, we can enhance our emotional well-being, lift our spirits, and find comfort or release in challenging times.

- Focus and Concentration: Certain types of music, such as instrumental or ambient tracks, can enhance focus and concentration. The absence of lyrics and rhythmic patterns can minimize distractions and create an environment conducive to deep work, studying, or engaging in tasks that require sustained attention. Specific frequencies, such as alpha or beta waves, can also be incorporated into music to stimulate alertness and mental clarity.

- Meditation and Mindfulness: Music is often used as a support tool for meditation and mindfulness practices. Gentle, ambient sounds, nature sounds, or repetitive patterns can serve as anchors, helping individuals stay present and focused during their meditation practice. Certain frequencies, such as theta or delta waves, are associated with deep states of relaxation and can facilitate a meditative state, promoting inner stillness and a sense of connectedness.

- Sleep Enhancement: Music has the potential to improve sleep quality and support a restful night's sleep. Slow, soothing melodies and nature sounds can create a conducive environment for relaxation and help individuals unwind before bedtime. Some frequencies, such as delta waves, are associated with deep sleep and can be incorporated into sleep music or guided sleep meditations to promote a more restorative sleep experience.
- Energetic Balance and Healing: Specific frequencies, such as the Solfeggio frequencies or the ancient Indian concept of "ragas," are believed to have healing properties and can help restore energetic balance within the body. These frequencies are thought to resonate with different energy centers or chakras and promote physical, emotional, and spiritual harmony. By immersing ourselves in music or soundscapes with these frequencies, we

can create an environment that supports energetic balance and healing.

It's important to note that individual responses to music and specific frequencies can vary. Each person may have unique preferences and sensitivities to different types of music. What promotes balance for one person may not have the same effect on another. It's essential to explore and experiment with different genres, styles, and frequencies to discover what resonates and supports your own physical and mental well-being.

By incorporating music and specific frequencies into our lives intentionally, we can tap into their transformative power and use them as tools for promoting physical and mental balance. Whether it's through active listening, engaging in music therapy, or creating personalized playlists, we have the opportunity to harness the therapeutic potential of music and sound to nurture our body and soul.

PEMF Therapy Explained

PEMF therapy, which stands for Pulsed Electromagnetic Field therapy, is a form of therapy that utilizes electromagnetic fields to promote healing and overall well-being. It involves the application of low-frequency pulsed electromagnetic waves to the body, either by using specialized devices or electromagnetic coils.

The basic principle behind PEMF therapy is that electromagnetic fields can interact with the body's cells and tissues, stimulating various biological processes. These electromagnetic pulses are thought to penetrate deep into the body, influencing the cells' electrical and magnetic properties.

PEMF therapy has been used for a variety of purposes, including pain management, tissue repair, and improving overall health. It is believed to work by increasing blood flow, reducing inflammation, and promoting cellular regeneration. This therapy is non-invasive and painless, and it can be applied to specific areas of the body or used in whole-body treatments.

It's important to note that while there is anecdotal evidence and some scientific research supporting the potential benefits of PEMF therapy, more rigorous studies are needed to establish its effectiveness for specific conditions. As with any therapy, it's advisable to consult with a healthcare professional before beginning PEMF treatment, especially if you have any underlying health conditions or are pregnant.

PEMF therapy works by applying low-frequency electromagnetic fields to the body, which interact with the body's cells and tissues. The exact mechanisms of how PEMF therapy works are not yet fully understood, but there are several proposed theories:

- Cellular Effects: PEMF therapy is believed to affect the electrical and magnetic properties of cells. It may induce tiny electrical currents in the cells, which can influence cellular signaling and communication. This, in turn, can impact various cellular processes such as metabolism, protein synthesis, and cell growth.
- Blood Flow and Circulation: PEMF therapy has been observed to increase blood flow and circulation in the treated area. Electromagnetic fields may stimulate the production of nitric oxide, a molecule that helps dilate blood vessels and improve blood flow.

Increased blood flow can deliver more oxygen and nutrients to the tissues while removing waste products, promoting healing and tissue repair.

- Anti-Inflammatory Effects: PEMF therapy has shown potential anti-inflammatory effects. It may help modulate the production of inflammatory molecules and immune responses, reducing inflammation in the body. By reducing inflammation, PEMF therapy can alleviate pain, swelling, and discomfort associated with various conditions.
- Calcium Ion Movement: Electromagnetic fields generated during PEMF therapy may influence the movement of calcium ions across cell membranes. Calcium ions play a crucial role in many cellular processes, including muscle contraction, nerve signaling, and gene expression. By modulating calcium ion movement, PEMF therapy can impact these cellular processes and potentially promote healing and tissue regeneration.
- Cellular Regeneration and Repair: PEMF therapy has been associated with increased cellular regeneration and repair. The electromagnetic fields may stimulate the production of proteins

involved in tissue repair and regeneration, promote cell proliferation, and accelerate the healing process. This can be beneficial for conditions involving injuries, fractures, and wounds.

It's important to note that the exact mechanisms of action for PEMF therapy are still being studied and researched. Different devices may use varying frequencies, intensities, and treatment durations, which can influence the therapeutic effects. The effectiveness of PEMF therapy may also depend on the specific condition being treated and individual factors. Therefore, it's advisable to consult with a healthcare professional or a qualified PEMF therapist for personalized guidance and treatment recommendations.

PEMF therapy has been associated with a range of potential benefits. While further research is needed to fully understand and validate these effects, here are some of the reported benefits of PEMF therapy:

- Pain Management: One of the primary uses of PEMF therapy is pain relief. It has been applied in various conditions, including chronic pain, arthritis, fibromyalgia, and musculoskeletal injuries. PEMF therapy may help alleviate pain by reducing inflammation, increasing blood circulation, and modulating pain perception. By promoting the release of endorphins, the body's natural painkillers, PEMF therapy can provide analgesic effects.

- Accelerated Healing: PEMF therapy is believed to enhance the body's natural healing processes. It can promote tissue repair, reduce recovery time, and improve overall healing outcomes. The electromagnetic fields stimulate cellular metabolism, increase protein synthesis, and enhance the production of factors involved in tissue regeneration. This can be beneficial for conditions such as fractures, wounds, sprains, and surgical incisions.
- Improved Sleep Quality: Many individuals report improved sleep quality after undergoing PEMF therapy. The therapy can help relax the body and mind, reduce stress levels, and promote a more restful sleep. By balancing neurotransmitters and influencing brainwave patterns, PEMF therapy may help regulate sleep cycles and alleviate sleep disturbances.

- Enhanced Physical Performance: PEMF therapy has been utilized by athletes and fitness enthusiasts to improve performance and enhance recovery. It may help optimize cellular function, increase energy production, and reduce muscle fatigue. By improving blood flow and oxygen delivery to muscles, PEMF therapy can enhance endurance, strength, and overall athletic performance.
- Reduced Inflammation: Chronic inflammation is implicated in various health conditions. PEMF therapy has shown potential in reducing inflammation by modulating immune responses and inhibiting the production of pro-inflammatory substances. By reducing inflammation, PEMF therapy can alleviate symptoms associated with conditions like arthritis, autoimmune disorders, and chronic inflammatory diseases.
- Bone Health and Density: PEMF therapy has been investigated for its effects on bone health. It may help improve bone density, increase calcium uptake, and enhance bone formation. This can be beneficial for individuals with

osteoporosis, osteoarthritis, or those recovering from fractures or orthopedic surgeries.

- Mental Wellness and Mood Enhancement: PEMF therapy has been associated with improvements in mental well-being and mood. The therapy may help regulate neurotransmitter levels, including serotonin and dopamine, which play key roles in mood regulation. By reducing stress, promoting relaxation, and improving sleep quality, PEMF therapy can contribute to a positive mental state.

Frequencies that Heal

PEMF therapy utilizes electromagnetic fields at specific frequencies to promote healing in humans. The choice of frequency in PEMF therapy depends on the desired therapeutic effect and the specific condition being treated. Here are some commonly used PEMF frequencies associated with healing benefits:

- Extremely Low Frequencies (ELF): Frequencies in the range of 1-100 Hz are often used in PEMF therapy. These frequencies are believed to mimic the natural electromagnetic signals present in the body. ELF frequencies have been associated with pain reduction, improved tissue repair, and anti-inflammatory effects. They are commonly used for general wellness, pain management, and promoting overall healing.

- Low Frequencies (LF): Frequencies between 1-1000 Hz are utilized in this range. Low frequencies are believed to stimulate cellular processes, enhance protein synthesis, and accelerate tissue regeneration. They have been used for various conditions such as bone fractures, wound healing, and musculoskeletal injuries. Frequencies in the range of 5-50 Hz are often employed for these purposes.

- Medium Frequencies (MF): Frequencies in the range of 1-10 kHz fall into the medium frequency range. MF frequencies are known for their deeper penetration into tissues compared to lower frequencies. They have been used to promote circulation, reduce pain and inflammation, and enhance cellular metabolism. MF frequencies are commonly employed for conditions such as osteoarthritis, neuropathic pain, and circulatory disorders.

- High Frequencies (HF): Frequencies above 10 kHz fall into the high-frequency range. HF frequencies are typically used for superficial tissue stimulation and wound healing. They have been associated with improved cell proliferation, increased oxygenation, and enhanced wound closure. Frequencies in the range of 10-100 kHz are often utilized for promoting healing in surface wounds, ulcers, and skin conditions.

At-Home PEMF Therapy

At-home PEMF therapy refers to the use of portable or consumer-grade PEMF devices for self-treatment in the comfort of one's own home. These devices are designed to provide convenient access to PEMF therapy without the need for frequent visits to a healthcare professional or specialized clinic. Here are some key points to consider regarding at-home PEMF therapy:

- Device Types: There are various types of at-home PEMF devices available on the market. These can include mat systems, localized applicators, handheld devices, and wearable devices. Mat systems are designed for whole-body treatment and are used by lying on or placing the mat on a specific area. Localized applicators target specific body parts or areas, while handheld and wearable devices offer more flexibility in terms of targeting different regions of the body.
- Ease of Use: At-home PEMF devices are typically designed to be user-friendly and easy to operate. They often come with pre-set programs or adjustable settings for selecting the desired frequency, intensity, and treatment duration. The devices may also provide guidance through display screens, control panels, or mobile applications.
- Treatment Duration and Frequency: The recommended treatment duration and frequency may vary depending on the device and the specific condition being treated. It's important to follow the

manufacturer's instructions and guidelines provided with the device. Generally, at-home PEMF therapy sessions can range from a few minutes to several hours, and treatments may be performed once or multiple times per day.

- Targeted Conditions: At-home PEMF therapy can be used for a variety of conditions, including pain management, muscle and joint issues, sports injuries, post-surgical recovery, and general wellness. However, it's important to note that the efficacy of at-home PEMF therapy for specific conditions may vary, and individual results can differ.
- Safety Considerations: While at-home PEMF devices are generally considered safe, it's important to follow the safety guidelines provided by the manufacturer. This includes using the device as directed, avoiding excessive or prolonged use, and consulting a healthcare professional if you have any underlying health conditions or concerns. Additionally, it's advisable to purchase devices from reputable manufacturers and ensure they meet safety and quality standards.

- Complementary Approach: At-home PEMF therapy is often used as a complementary approach alongside other conventional medical treatments. It's important to view it as a part of an overall wellness plan and to consult with a healthcare professional for a comprehensive evaluation and treatment recommendations.

It's worth noting that while at-home PEMF therapy provides convenience and accessibility, it's essential to be informed and make informed decisions regarding device selection, usage, and treatment parameters. Consulting with a healthcare professional or a PEMF therapist can provide personalized guidance, ensure safety, and optimize the potential benefits of at-home PEMF therapy.

Qi Coils and Other Products

Qi Life Store's Qi Machine is a revolutionary product developed in collaboration with a team of dedicated researchers. Its purpose is to transform the way we approach meditation by introducing groundbreaking innovations.

The centerpiece of this innovation is the Qi Coils, an advanced portable PEMF (Pulsed Electromagnetic Field) system. By utilizing a combination of unique sound and electromagnetic waves, the Qi Coils guide the body and mind to achieve optimal performance and well-being.

The Qi Coils are specifically designed to create electromagnetic fields that produce accompanying sounds, working in tandem to elevate human consciousness to levels beyond the ordinary. Through this harmonious fusion of electromagnetic and auditory stimulation, the Qi Machine aids in removing negativity from the body while absorbing positive energy. This process promotes inner harmony, clarity, and a sense of tranquility similar to the effects of meditation, resulting in a calm state of being for the body, mind, and spirit.

At the core of the Qi Coils system lies its ability to transmit electromagnetic frequencies through a mobile app via a patent-pending magnetic coil. The Qi Coils consist of a Yin Coil and a Yang Coil, each playing a crucial role in their unique operation. These coils effectively clear away negative energy and facilitate the attraction of positive energy, offering an easier path to calming the mind and discovering true inner peace.

Using specific sounds and frequencies, Qi Coils work in synergy to enhance meditation practices, boost personal energy levels, facilitate abundance attraction and manifestation, rejuvenate the body and mind, and expand the overall state of consciousness. By converting electrical signals into magnetic wave signals, the Qi Machine generates a wide range of frequencies. Amplified and transmitted as energy waves, these frequency signals penetrate every cell in the body, delivering their benefits to any desired area. Consequently, the Qi Machine serves as the world's first Neuro-Programming Magnetic Energy Emitter, effectively promoting physical and mental well-being.

To utilize the Qi Machine, one must connect the Qi Coil to a smartphone and log into the Qi Coil App. When a chosen frequency plays through the Qi Coil, it generates a powerful electromagnetic field with a reach of approximately three feet. This field acts upon the body's "biological field," harmonizing and renewing it over time. The result is a positive and healthy infusion for both the body and mind.

The unique vortex angle of the Qi Coil enables 360-degree directional electromagnetic regeneration, known as PEMF (Pulsed Electromagnetic Field), targeting any specific area of the body. This functionality stimulates cell regeneration within bones, tissues, and nerve cells, thereby contributing to overall physical rejuvenation and well-being.

All things considered, Qi Coil is the most versatile option for at-home PEMF therapy. This all comes down to the countless offerings that cater to pretty much all your needs. It has something for everybody.

It is better than other rife machines due to the simple fact that it packs the features that matter. Other rife machines may have lights and other design features that make them stand out, but they are unneeded. They only generate radio frequencies whereas Qi Coils can do a lot more than basic radio frequencies. In fact, it offers over 150,000 frequencies to choose from with different effects. So, you are not starved for options here.

Not to mention, the pricing for Qi Coils can be very low if you are just starting out whereas other rife machines require a lot of investment which can be discouraging for people who want to experience the healing power of frequencies firsthand.

If you are unsure about at-home PEMF therapy and healing through sound, you can invest a small amount of cash into a very basic Qi Coil setup and then expand your repertoire from there. And there is a lot of room for expansion so you can explore the power of sound healing at your own pace.

If you are just starting out and experimenting, you can hardly go wrong with Qi Coil Mini. Marked as "entry-level", this product offers a modest yet versatile number of features such as helping you relieve pain, regenerate, relax, sleep, de-stress, and meditate.

If you are happy with your purchase and want to explore more of what Qi Coil has to offer, you have two options. If you are on the move and want to tap into this healing power on the go, the 3S Quantanium variant is the best way to go. It features a tri-crystal chamber toroidal crystalline orgone base, Yin Yang Vortex, Bluetooth capability, basic frequencies you would get from the Mini variant, 24 Master Frequencies, and over 800 Quantum Frequencies Transformation Course with a number of other accessories. The range is 11 feet for each coil and it contains 3 Quantanium crystals.

But if you want the best from your Qi Coil, you can go for the MAX Quantanium. It is heavier than the 3S Quantanium, making it a better option for stationary use. With this, you get 20 feet radius for each coil and within it, you get 6 Quantanium Crystals. The base is hexa-crystal chamber crystalline orgone and all the features from the 3S Quantanium.

On top of all this, there are resonant consoles and other products to help you.

There are, of course, other products on the market if you want to explore other options:

- Resonant Wave: A close competitor with similar features and 170 square feet in range, but it is also incredibly expensive.
- Healy: A slightly more expensive product with not as many features. Other than the fact that contact is needed, it only comes with 30 frequencies.
- Muse: The price is about the same as the Qi Coil Mini, but it requires contact just like the Healy, and lacks important features to help you tap into the healing

power of frequencies. Plus, it does not come with any preset frequencies.

- iMRS 2000: Contact is also needed here and on top of being quite expensive and difficult to set up, it also lacks important features that make the Qi Coil stand out.
- Bemer: Also very expensive and difficult to set up, it comes with one base frequency and not many other innovative features that the Qi Coil offers.

Chapter 5: The Future of Sound Healing

The resurgence of interest in healing frequencies reflects a broader shift towards integrative and holistic approaches to health and wellness. As people seek natural and non-invasive methods to support their well-being, the power of sound and vibrations offers a captivating avenue for exploration. Whether through binaural beats, solfeggio frequencies, or sound baths, the ancient wisdom of sound therapy continues to inspire and captivate individuals, igniting a renewed curiosity in the potential of healing frequencies to promote balance, rejuvenation, and overall vitality in modern times.

While the scientific understanding of the precise mechanisms behind the therapeutic effects of healing frequencies is still evolving, there is growing research in this field. Studies have shown promising results, suggesting that sound therapy can positively impact various aspects of health, including stress reduction, pain management, sleep improvement, and emotional well-being. Additionally, the subjective experiences and anecdotal reports from individuals who have incorporated healing frequencies into their lives provide further support for their potential benefits.

As more and more people start to understand and realize the healing power of sound healing, it is very possible that sound healing becomes commonplace in the healthcare industry.

Potential Integration of Sound Healing into Maintaining Healthcare

The integration of sound healing into mainstream healthcare is an area that is gaining attention and recognition for its potential therapeutic benefits. Sound healing involves the use of sound frequencies, vibrations, and music to promote relaxation, reduce stress, and support the body's natural healing processes. Here are some points that elaborate on the potential integration of sound healing into mainstream healthcare:

1. Stress Reduction and Relaxation: Sound healing techniques, such as listening to calming music or participating in sound baths, have been found to induce a state of deep relaxation and reduce stress. Stress reduction is a crucial component of overall health and well-being, and integrating sound healing practices into mainstream healthcare can provide additional tools to address this common concern.

2. Pain Management: Sound therapy has shown promising results in managing pain. Certain sound frequencies and vibrations have been found to stimulate the release of endorphins, the body's natural pain-relieving chemicals. Sound healing modalities, including binaural beats and specific sound frequencies, can potentially be used alongside conventional pain management techniques to enhance pain relief and improve overall patient comfort.

3. Emotional Well-being: Sound healing can positively impact emotional well-being by promoting feelings of calmness, improving mood, and reducing symptoms of anxiety and depression.

Incorporating sound healing practices into mainstream healthcare can offer complementary approaches to support mental health, alongside traditional therapies such as counseling or medication.

4. Enhanced Mind-Body Connection: Sound healing practices often involve deep listening and mindfulness, which can help individuals develop a stronger mind-body connection. This increased awareness of the body's sensations, emotions, and energetic flow can contribute to a more holistic approach to healthcare, fostering self-awareness and self-care.

5. Complementary Therapy: Sound healing can serve as a complementary therapy alongside conventional medical treatments. It can be integrated into various healthcare settings, including hospitals, clinics, rehabilitation centers, and wellness centers. By incorporating sound healing techniques into treatment plans, healthcare providers can offer a more comprehensive and patient-centered approach to care.

6. **Improved Patient Experience:** Integrating sound healing into mainstream healthcare can enhance the patient experience. It can create a more soothing and supportive environment for patients, reducing anxiety and improving overall satisfaction. Sound healing practices can be incorporated into waiting areas, treatment rooms, and pre- and post-procedure settings to promote relaxation and create a sense of calm.

7. **Research and Evidence-Based Practice:** As sound healing gains recognition, more research is being conducted to explore its effectiveness and benefits. Evidence-based studies can provide valuable insights into the specific applications, protocols, and outcomes of sound healing in various healthcare contexts. This research can contribute to the integration of sound healing practices into mainstream healthcare, ensuring that they are implemented in a safe, evidence-based manner.

8. **Training and Education:** The integration of sound healing into mainstream healthcare would require training and

education for healthcare providers to ensure their competency and understanding of sound healing techniques. Continuing education programs, workshops, and certifications can help healthcare professionals gain the necessary skills to incorporate sound healing into their practice.

While the integration of sound healing into mainstream healthcare is still evolving, its potential benefits and growing body of research suggest that it can be a valuable addition to conventional medical approaches. Collaboration between sound healing practitioners and healthcare professionals can contribute to the development of comprehensive treatment plans that address both the physical and emotional aspects of patient care.

Emerging Research

Emerging research and technological advancements in sound healing are paving the way for exciting developments and expanding our understanding of the profound effects of sound on our well-being. As science and technology continue to progress, we gain deeper insights into the therapeutic potential of sound and its applications in various healing modalities. Here are some key areas of research and technological advancements in sound healing:

1. Brainwave Entrainment: Brainwave entrainment is a technique that uses sound frequencies to synchronize the brainwaves with external stimuli. Research has shown that specific sound frequencies, such as binaural beats or isochronic tones, can influence brainwave activity and induce desired states of consciousness, such as relaxation, focus, or sleep. This technology is being further refined and integrated into audio programs and wearable devices for personal use.

2. Sound Therapy Devices: Technological advancements have led to the development of specialized sound therapy devices. These devices utilize a variety of sound frequencies, including specific healing frequencies and harmonics, to deliver therapeutic effects. Examples include sound healing

tables, chairs, mats, and pillows that use vibrations and resonances to promote relaxation and balance in the body.

3. Sound Analysis and Mapping: Advanced sound analysis techniques are being used to study the effects of sound on the body and mind. This research involves mapping the frequencies and vibrations of sound and their impact on specific areas of the body or brain. Through this analysis, researchers are gaining insights into how different sound frequencies can influence physiological functions, brain activity, and emotional states.

4. Soundscapes and Sonic Environments: The study of soundscapes and sonic environments focuses on how different soundscapes can impact human health and well-being. Researchers are exploring the effects of natural sounds, such as flowing water, birdsong, or gentle winds, on stress reduction, cognitive performance, and emotional well-being. Additionally, advancements in virtual reality and immersive audio technologies allow individuals to

experience curated soundscapes for therapeutic purposes.

5. Sound and Cellular Biology: Sound healing research is also delving into the cellular and molecular effects of sound vibrations on the body. Studies have shown that sound can influence cellular activities, gene expression, and cellular signaling pathways. This field of research aims to understand the mechanisms through which sound vibrations can promote cellular healing and regeneration.

6. Personalized Sound Healing: Advancements in technology are enabling personalized sound healing experiences. With the use of biofeedback devices, genetic testing, or artificial intelligence algorithms, sound healing programs can be tailored to individual needs and preferences. This approach takes into account an individual's unique physiological and psychological characteristics to deliver customized sound frequencies and compositions for optimal therapeutic outcomes.

7. Integration with Other Modalities: Sound healing is being integrated with other healing modalities, such as meditation, energy work, and mindfulness practices. Combining sound with practices like guided imagery, breathwork, or Reiki amplifies the overall therapeutic effects and enhances the mind-body connection.

As research and technology continue to advance, we can expect further breakthroughs in sound healing. These advancements hold the potential to revolutionize healthcare by providing innovative, non-invasive, and accessible approaches to support physical, mental, and emotional well-being. With ongoing exploration and open-mindedness, we will continue to uncover the extraordinary potential of sound as a powerful tool for healing and transformation.

Chapter 6:
Practical Exercises

Here comes the fun part. You have learned much about the healing powers of sounds, but how exactly do you tap into this? We will talk about all of that in this chapter.

How to Implement PEMF Therapy at Home

Implementing PEMF therapy at home involves a few key steps to ensure safe and effective treatment. Here's a general guide on how to implement PEMF therapy at home:

- Research and select a device: Begin by researching different at-home PEMF devices available on the market. Consider factors such as device type (mat, localized applicator, handheld, wearable), intended use, user reviews, and safety features. Choose a device that suits your specific needs and meets your preferences.

- Read the instructions: Carefully read the manufacturer's instructions and user manual provided with the device. Familiarize yourself with the device's features, settings, recommended treatment protocols, and safety precautions. It's important to understand how to properly operate and maintain the device.

- Find a suitable treatment area: Find a suitable area in your home where you can comfortably perform PEMF therapy. Ensure that you have enough space to lie down, place a mat, or position the device as required. Make sure the area is clean, tidy, and promote a sense of calmness and relaxation.

- Set up the device: Set up the PEMF device according to the manufacturer's instructions. This may involve connecting power cords, attaching applicators or electrodes, or adjusting settings such as frequency, intensity, and treatment duration. Follow the specific guidelines provided for your device.

- Prepare for treatment: Prepare yourself for the treatment session. This may involve removing any metal objects or jewelry that could interfere with the electromagnetic fields. Ensure you are in a relaxed and comfortable position, either lying down or sitting, depending on the device and treatment area.
- Start treatment: Begin the PEMF therapy session according to the recommended settings. Follow the treatment duration and frequency suggested by the manufacturer. During the session, relax and allow the device to emit the pulsed electromagnetic fields while you remain in a comfortable position.
- Observe safety precautions: Adhere to the safety precautions provided with the device. Avoid exceeding the recommended treatment duration or intensity levels. If you experience any discomfort or adverse effects during the treatment, stop using the device and consult a healthcare professional.
- Maintain consistency: Consistency is important for obtaining potential benefits from PEMF therapy. Depending on the condition being treated, you may need to perform PEMF therapy sessions

regularly. Follow the recommended treatment schedule and duration for your specific condition.

- Regular maintenance: Properly maintain and care for your PEMF device. Follow the cleaning and maintenance instructions provided by the manufacturer to ensure the device's longevity and optimal performance.

- Consult a healthcare professional: It's always advisable to consult with a healthcare professional or a PEMF therapist before starting at-home PEMF therapy, especially if you have any underlying health conditions or concerns. They can provide personalized guidance, recommend specific treatment protocols, and ensure the therapy complements your overall healthcare plan.

Remember, the specific implementation of PEMF therapy may vary depending on the device and the condition being treated. Always refer to the device's instructions and seek professional guidance for your individual circumstances.

How to Apply Frequencies at Home

Applying healing frequencies into daily life can involve incorporating various practices and activities that promote well-being and support the body's natural healing processes. While the specific frequencies used in PEMF therapy are not typically applied directly in daily life, here are some general steps you can take to support healing and overall wellness:

- Establish a routine: Create a daily routine that includes dedicated time for self-care and well-being. This routine can consist of activities that promote relaxation, stress reduction, and physical and mental health.

- Mindful breathing and meditation: Incorporate mindful breathing exercises and meditation into your daily routine. Mindful breathing can actually be practiced pretty much everywhere and it is a quick way to reduce stress, heighten focus, and instill a sense of calmness. Focus on deep, slow breaths, and find a quiet and comfortable space for meditation.

- Physical exercise: Engage in regular physical exercise that suits your fitness level and preferences. Physical activity helps improve circulation, release endorphins, and support overall physical and mental well-being. Choose activities you enjoy, whether it's walking, jogging, yoga, dancing, or any other form of exercise.

- Healthy nutrition: Pay attention to your diet and nourish your body with healthy, nutrient-rich foods. That means consuming a variety of fruits, veggies, whole grains, etc. Try to be as natural as possible. Not to mention, make sure to drink enough water throughout the day. If you feel thirsty, you are already dehydrated, so drink some water as soon as possible.

- Adequate sleep: Doctors recommend 7-9 hours of sleep and this is non-negotiable. Get quality sleep by switching off electronics an hour before bed and spend that time reading, meditating, or relaxing instead. Doing so promotes sleep quality. Moreover, have a consistent sleep routine and schedule. Establish a relaxing bedtime routine to signal to your body that it's time to wind down. That means, have a set of activities that you go through before bed to help you relax. Going to sleep at regular hours also go a long way in helping you sleep and wake up at precise hours. With enough practice, you can wake up a minute before the alarm goes off. Most importantly, the bedroom should also promote sleep and relaxation. That means, the bedroom needs to be cool, dark, and quiet.

- Stress management: Practice stress management techniques to reduce the negative impact of stress on your body and mind. This can include activities such as journaling, practicing mindfulness, engaging in hobbies, spending time in nature, or seeking support from a therapist or support group.

- Social connections: Foster healthy social connections with friends, family, and the community. Engage in activities that promote positive social interactions, such as joining clubs or groups with shared interests, participating in community events, or simply spending quality time with loved ones.

- Rest and relaxation: Make time for rest and relaxation throughout the day. Incorporate activities that help you unwind, such as taking breaks, engaging in hobbies, listening to soothing music, practicing deep breathing exercises, or enjoying a bath.

- Regular check-ups: Schedule regular check-ups with healthcare professionals to monitor your overall health and address any potential issues promptly. It's important to have a comprehensive evaluation of your physical and mental well-being to ensure early detection and appropriate interventions if needed.

- Continuous learning: Stay informed and engaged in learning about health, wellness, and self-care. Stay updated on the latest research and evidence-based practices that can support your healing journey. This can include reading books, listening to podcasts, attending workshops, or consulting with healthcare professionals.

Implementing Healing Frequencies

In the fast-paced and often demanding modern world, prioritizing self-care becomes crucial for maintaining our physical, emotional, and mental well-being. One powerful way to integrate self-care techniques into our daily lives is by incorporating healing frequencies. Here are numerous ways you can implement self-care techniques with healing frequencies into your daily routine:

1. Morning ritual: Begin your day with a few moments of calmness and intention. Sit quietly and listen to a guided meditation or soothing music embedded with healing frequencies. Allow the vibrations to gently awaken your mind and set a positive tone for the day ahead.

2. Mindful breathing: Throughout the day, take regular breaks to focus on your breath. As you inhale deeply, visualize healing frequencies entering your body, cleansing and revitalizing every cell. Exhale, releasing any tension or negativity. This simple practice can be

done anywhere, promoting relaxation and rejuvenation.

3. Sound bath: Set aside time for a dedicated sound bath session. Create a tranquil environment, either by playing recorded sound healing tracks or using instruments like singing bowls or chimes. Immerse yourself in the soothing vibrations, allowing them to wash over you and restore balance.

4. Music therapy: Incorporate healing frequency-infused music into your daily life. Whether during work, chores, or relaxation time, listen to uplifting melodies that resonate with your desired healing goals. Let the harmonious frequencies envelop you, promoting a sense of peace and well-being.

5. Walking in nature: Combine the healing power of nature with sound healing. Take a mindful walk in a park or natural setting, using headphones to listen to nature-inspired soundscapes or guided meditations infused with healing frequencies. Allow the sounds of nature

and healing vibrations to ground and rejuvenate you.

6. Energetic clearing: Use sound frequencies to cleanse and balance your energy. Explore practices like chanting, toning, or using sound instruments to clear stagnant energy from your aura and chakras. Allow the vibrations to realign and restore your energetic system.

7. Evening wind-down: Create a soothing wind-down routine before bed. Dim the lights, play calming music with healing frequencies, and engage in relaxation exercises. Focus on releasing the day's stress and tension, preparing your mind and body for restorative sleep.

8. Breathing with intent: Before sleep, practice deep breathing exercises while visualizing healing frequencies enveloping your entire being. Inhale healing energy, and with each exhale, release any physical or mental discomfort. This practice promotes relaxation and prepares you for a restful night's sleep.

9. Healing baths: Transform your bathing routine into a healing ritual. Add Epsom salts, essential oils, or crystals known for their healing properties to your bathwater. Enhance the experience by playing sound healing tracks or guided meditations designed for relaxation and rejuvenation.

10. Intentional listening: Throughout the day, consciously choose to listen to music or soundscapes that resonate with healing frequencies. Whether during work, exercise, or leisure time, let the sounds you surround yourself with support your well-being and uplift your mood.

Remember, self-care is a personal journey, and it's important to explore and find what resonates with you. Experiment with different techniques and find the ones that bring you the most comfort and joy. By integrating healing frequencies into your daily life, you can cultivate a deeper sense of well-being, balance, and harmony, supporting your holistic health journey.

Meditation and Exercise

Guided meditations and exercises for self-healing and balance are powerful tools for promoting overall well-being and supporting the body's natural healing processes. These practices can be enhanced by incorporating at-home PEMF therapy, which can further elevate their effectiveness. Here's an elaboration on these topics:

1. Guided meditations and exercises for self-healing and balance: Guided meditations and exercises are structured practices that involve focusing the mind, regulating breathing, and promoting relaxation. They can help reduce stress, increase self-awareness, and facilitate healing on physical, mental, and emotional levels. These practices often incorporate visualization, affirmation, and mindfulness techniques to support the body's healing processes and restore balance.

2. Integration of at-home PEMF therapy: At-home PEMF therapy involves using portable PEMF devices to apply pulsed electromagnetic fields to the body.

When combined with guided meditations and exercises, PEMF therapy can enhance their effectiveness in several ways:

a) Deepening relaxation: PEMF therapy has been reported to induce a deep sense of relaxation and calm. By using PEMF therapy in conjunction with guided meditations, individuals may experience a deeper state of relaxation, allowing them to more effectively release tension, and stress, and promote self-healing.

b) Amplifying energy flow: Guided meditations often involve visualization and focusing on the flow of energy within the body. PEMF therapy has the potential to stimulate and enhance the body's energy flow, aiding in the balancing and harmonizing of the body's energetic systems.

c) Supporting cellular health: PEMF therapy is believed to promote cellular health and optimize cellular functioning. When combined with guided meditations and exercises, which focus on self-healing and balance, PEMF therapy can provide an additional layer of support to the body's cellular processes, potentially enhancing the body's ability to heal and restore itself.

d) Promoting mind-body connection: Both guided meditations and PEMF therapy encourage a stronger mind-body connection. Guided meditations facilitate awareness of the body's sensations, emotions, and energetic flow, while PEMF therapy influences cellular and physiological processes. Combining these practices can deepen the mind-body connection, allowing individuals to engage more fully in their self-healing journey.

3. Integration techniques: Here are some ways to integrate at-home PEMF therapy with guided meditations and exercises:

a) Set the environment: Create a peaceful and comfortable space for your practice, free from distractions. Set up your PEMF device according to the manufacturer's instructions and have it ready for use.

b) Pre-session PEMF therapy: Before starting a guided meditation or exercise, you can incorporate a short session of PEMF therapy to relax and prepare the body. Lie or sit comfortably with the PEMF device placed appropriately, and allow yourself to relax and enter a calm state.

c) Combined practice: You can choose guided meditations or exercises specifically designed to be practiced with PEMF therapy. Look for guided meditations or programs that incorporate energetic healing, visualization, or affirmations that align with your specific self-healing goals.

d) Post-session PEMF therapy: Following a guided meditation or exercise, you can continue the healing process by utilizing PEMF therapy. Allow the PEMF device to support your body's relaxation and recovery, promoting the integration of the practices into your system.

4. Personalization and professional guidance: It's important to personalize your approach and choose guided meditations, exercises, and PEMF therapy settings that resonate with your specific needs and goals. Additionally, if you have any underlying health conditions or concerns, or if you're unsure about the appropriate use of PEMF therapy, it's advisable to consult with a healthcare professional or a PEMF therapist who can provide personalized guidance and recommendations.

Conclusion

And there you have it. I have shared with you everything you need to know to unlock your full potential as you set out on this journey toward balance and profound healing. Of course, there is still much to learn, I implore you to explore the potential of sound healing and embrace the transformative power of vibrations in your own journey towards physical and mental well-being.

Though these practices you see here have yet to be fully adopted by contemporary medicine, there is a good chance that they are brought into the spotlight. Their potentials are there and despite their healing powers, not a lot of people know about this. But before long, the future where the harmonious melodies of healing frequencies resonate in hospitals, clinics, and even within the sanctuaries of our homes becomes a reality.

Embrace the symphony of guided meditations and exercises that nourish your soul and cultivate inner balance. Allow the vibrations to ripple through your being, resonating with every cell and fiber of your existence. With each breath, become attuned to the sacred rhythm of life, the symphony that permeates all creation.

As we explored the interplay of sound and consciousness, we uncovered the profound potential of Qi energy. Embrace this remarkable fusion of science and spirituality, where pulsating electromagnetic fields merge with the frequencies of your soul. It is through this integration that we elevate our self-healing practices, transcending the limitations of the physical realm.

In this era of awakening, we stand poised to unlock the full potential of sound healing in our lives. Embrace the opportunity to experiment, to immerse yourself in the healing vibrations that resonate with your unique essence. Let the waves of sound carry you to realms of tranquility, where your spirit soars and your body rejuvenates.

The power of sound healing is a sacred gift bestowed upon us. Seek out the guidance of experts, delve into the profound wisdom of ancient traditions, and create a symphony of self-healing that resonates with your very soul.

Together, let us educate and forge a future where the profound impact of sound and vibrations is recognized, where mainstream healthcare embraces the symphony of healing frequencies, and where the integration of science and spirituality paves the way for a world of profound physical and mental well-being.

May the melodies of healing embrace you, may the vibrations of transformation uplift you, and may your journey toward wholeness be illuminated by the symphony of sound.

Imprint

Important Notice:

The information contained in this book is for informational purposes only and under no circumstances should be considered a substitute for professional advice or treatment by trained and credentialed physicians. It does not include any recommendations regarding specific diagnostic or therapeutic procedures. The contents should never be construed as a request for self-treatment or as a basis for self-diagnosis and self-medication. The information reflects only the opinion of the author. The author makes no warranty, express or implied, as to the nature or accuracy of the contents.

Should any content of the book violate applicable law, the author requests immediate notification. The content in question will then be removed or changed immediately.

Liability for links

The book contains links to external websites of third parties, on whose contents we have no influence. Therefore, we cannot assume any liability for these external contents. The respective provider or operator of the pages is always responsible for the content of the linked pages. The linked pages were checked for possible legal violations at the time of linking. Illegal contents were not recognizable at the time of linking. However, a permanent control of the contents of the linked pages is not reasonable without concrete evidence of a violation of the law. If we become aware of any infringements, we will remove such links immediately.